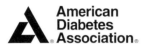American
Diabetes
Association

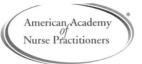American Academy
of
Nurse Practitioners

DIABETES READY REFERENCE

for Nurse Practitioners

....

Clear, concise guidelines for effective patient care

....

Diagnosis • Monitoring
Insulin Therapy • Oral Medications
Nutrition • Exercise • Complications
Surgery & Hospitalization

Director, Book Publishing, Abe Ogden; *Acquisitions Editor,* Victor Van Beuren; *Managing Editor,* Greg Guthrie; *Editor,* Rebekah Renshaw; *Writer,* IMPACT Health Communications, LLC; *Production Manager,* Melissa Sprott; *Composition,* ADA; *Cover Design,* Koncept, Inc.; *Printer,* Thomson-Shore, Inc.

Printed in the United States of America
3 5 7 9 10 8 6 4 2

The suggestions and information contained in this publication are generally consistent with the Clinical Practice Recommendations and other policies of the American Diabetes Association, but they do not represent the policy or position of the Association or any of its boards or committees. Reasonable steps have been taken to ensure the accuracy of the information presented. However, the American Diabetes Association cannot ensure the safety or efficacy of any product or service described in this publication. Individuals are advised to consult a clinician or other appropriate health care professional before undertaking any diet or exercise program or taking any medication referred to in this publication. Professionals must use and apply their own professional judgment, experience, and training and should not rely solely on the information contained in this publication before prescribing any diet, exercise, or medication. The American Diabetes Association—its officers, directors, employees, volunteers, and members—assumes no responsibility or liability for personal or other injury, loss, or damage that may result from the suggestions or information in this publication.

The information contained in this publication is generally consistent with the standards of care accepted at the time of publication. Health care is constantly changing, as new research and clinical experience support changes in recommendations. Healthcare professionals must use and apply their own professional judgment, experience, and training and should not rely solely on the information contained in this publication before prescribing any diet, exercise, or medication. Readers should verify the information with other sources and carefully consider the applicability to individual patients. The American Academy of Nurse Practitioners cannot ensure the safety or efficacy of any recommendation described in this publication and assumes no responsibility or liability for personal or other injury, loss, or damage that may result from the suggestions or information in this publication.

♾ The paper in this publication meets the requirements of the ANSI Standard Z39.48-1992 (permanence of paper).

ADA titles may be purchased for business or promotional use or for special sales. To purchase more than 50 copies of this book at a discount, or for custom editions of this book with your logo, contact the American Diabetes Association at the address below, at booksales@diabetes.org, or by calling 703-299-2046.

American Diabetes Association
1701 North Beauregard Street
Alexandria, Virginia 22311

DOI: 10.2337/9781580404464

Library of Congress Cataloging-in-Publication Data

Diabetes ready reference guide for nurse practitioners / by American Diabetes Association and American Academy of Nurse Practitioners.
    p. ; cm.
 Includes bibliographical references and index.
 ISBN 978-1-58040-446-4 (alk. paper)
 I. American Diabetes Association. II. American Academy of Nurse Practitioners.
 [DNLM: 1. Diabetes Mellitus--Handbooks. 2. Diabetes Mellitus--Nurses' Instruction. 3. Nurse Practitioners. WK 39]
 LCClassification not assigned
 616.4'62--dc23
                    2011030867

Contents

Acknowledgments

The American Diabetes Association gratefully acknowledges the following contributors to this book who shared their professional expertise and experience in this subject matter: Amanda Crowe, MA, MPH; Jane Kapustin, PhD, CRNP, BC-ADM, FAANP; Jane Jeffrie Seley, DNP, MPH, MSN, BC-ADM, CDE; Kathryn Mulcahy, RN, MSN, CDE, and Terry Lumber, APRN, CNS, MSN, BC-ADM, CDE.

Pathophysiology of Diabetes

I. DEFINITION OF DIABETES

A. Diabetes is a chronic metabolic disorder in which the body cannot metabolize carbohydrates, fats, and proteins because of defects in insulin secretion and/or action of insulin.

B. The chronic hyperglycemia of diabetes is associated with long-term damage, dysfunction, and failure of various organs, especially the eyes, kidneys, nerves, heart, and blood vessels.

C. Diabetes is classified into three primary types, which are different disease entities but share the symptoms and complications of hyperglycemia (high blood glucose).

D. Prediabetes is a degree of hyperglycemia that may precede type 2 diabetes and that increases risk for future diabetes and cardiovascular disease.

II. TYPE 1 DIABETES: BETA CELL DESTRUCTION, ABSOLUTE LACK OF INSULIN

A. Causes
1. Genetic predisposition
2. Environmental exposure: virus, toxin, stress
3. Autoimmune reaction: β-cells that produce insulin in the pancreas are destroyed. When 80–90% of the β-cells are destroyed, overt symptoms occur. 20% of patients have other autoimmune disorders, such as hypothyroidism, celiac disease, etc.

B. Characteristics
1. Usually occurs before 30 years of age, but can occur at any age. More than 50% cases are adults.
2. Abrupt onset of signs and symptoms of hyperglycemia: increased thirst and hunger, frequent urination, weight loss, and fatigue
3. Ketosis prone (typically type 1 diabetes)

C. Treatment
1. Insulin by injection with syringes or pump
2. Symlin (pramlintide acetate) as an adjunct to insulin

3. Medical nutrition therapy
4. Physical activity
5. Diabetes self-management education
6. Continuous glucose monitoring, self-monitoring of blood glucose and ketones

III. TYPE 2 DIABETES: RELATIVE INSULIN DEFICIENCY WITH ACCOMPANYING INSULIN RESISTANCE

A. Causes

1. Insulin resistance: less able to utilize insulin that the body makes because of cellular defects; glucose is less able to be absorbed properly into cells for fuel.
2. Decreased insulin secretion: β-cells in pancreas do not secrete enough insulin in response to rising glucose levels.
3. Excess production of glucose from the liver: result of insulin resistance and defective insulin secretory response, inability to regulate glucagon production; dawn phenomenon (see Glossary) is an example.

B. Characteristics

1. Usually occurs after 45 years of age, but can occur in children and early adulthood
2. Increased prevalence in some ethnic groups, e.g., African Americans, Latinos, Native Americans, Asian Americans, and Pacific Islanders
3. Strong genetic predisposition
4. Frequently overweight or obese at diagnosis
5. Not prone to ketoacidosis until late in course or with prolonged hyperglycemia
6. May or may not have symptoms of hyperglycemia
7. May also have blurred vision, delayed healing, numbness and tingling of the hands and feet, recurring yeast infection
8. 20% have established microvascular complications at diagnosis

C. Treatment

1. Meal planning/weight management/weight loss
2. Exercise/increased physical activity
3. Oral hypoglycemic/antihyperglycemic agents, insulin sensitizers, and/or insulin, other injectables (incretins, synthetic amylin)
4. Diabetes self-management education
5. Self-monitoring of blood glucose, continuous glucose monitoring
6. Treatment of comorbid conditions (e.g., hypertension, lipid abnormalities)

IV. GESTATIONAL DIABETES MELLITUS (GDM):

Glucose intolerance that develops during pregnancy and typically resolves with delivery, occurs in about 7% of all pregnancies or about 200,000/yr.

A. Causes and risk factors
   1. Insulin resistance due to pregnancy
   2. Overweight and obesity
   3. Genetic predisposition (being overweight or obese at time of pregnancy)

B. Characteristics
   1. Carbohydrate intolerance identified by screening those at risk during pregnancy (see page 7)
   2. Usually asymptomatic condition
   3. Strong risk factor for later development of type 2

C. Treatment
   1. Meal planning: Provide adequate calories without hyperglycemia or ketonemia, often divided into meals and snacks to space carbohydrate intake.
   2. Exercise: program that does not cause fetal distress, contractions, or hypertension (>130/80 mmHg)
   3. Weight management
   4. Medications:
      a. Insulin: Consider if unable to consistently maintain plasma glucose ≤90 mg/dl (≤5.0 mmol/l) fasting and ≤120 mg/dl (≤6.7 mmol/l) 1–2 hours postprandial.
      b. Oral agents: Glyburide, metformin are sometimes used (not recommended by the ADA).
   5. Self-monitoring
      a. Blood glucose: required to determine effectiveness of treatment and possible need for insulin. Glucose should be checked fasting and 1–2 hours postprandially.

Diagnosis of Diabetes

I. CRITERIA FOR DIAGNOSIS

A. Type 1 and type 2 diabetes

1. Nonpregnant adults

   a. Casual plasma glucose ≥200 mg/dl (≥11.1 mmol/l) plus classic symptoms

   OR

   Fasting plasma glucose (FPG) ≥126 mg/dl (≥7.0 mmol/l)

   OR

   2-hour plasma glucose (PG) ≥200 mg/dl (≥11.1 mmol/l) on 75-g oral glucose tolerance test (OGTT)

   OR

   A1C ≥ 6.5% using standardized lab method. A1C not accurate in anemia or hemoglobinopathies

   b. Each of the last three tests should be confirmed by an additional test on a subsequent day unless unequivocal hyperglycemia exists. This should be the same test (e.g., two FPGs or two A1Cs).

   c. OGTT rarely needed to diagnose type 1 diabetes

2. Children

   a. Same as for nonpregnant adults (see above)

   b. OGTT contraindicated in infants and young children

B. Gestational diabetes mellitus (GDM)

1. Perform a 75-g OGTT, with plasma glucose measurement fasting and at 1 and 2 h, at 24–28 weeks of gestation in women not previously diagnosed with overt diabetes. The OGTT should be performed in the morning after an overnight fast of at least 8 h. The diagnosis of GDM is made when any of the following plasma glucose values are exceeded:

   Fasting ≥92 mg/dl (5.1 mmol/l)
   1 h ≥180 mg/dl (10.0 mmol/l)
   2 h ≥53 mg/dl (8.5 mmol/l)

C. Pre-diabetes

1. Impaired fasting glucose (IFG): FPG ≥100 mg/dl (≥5.6 mmol/l) and <126 mg/dl (<7.0 mmol/l)

2. Impaired glucose tolerance (IGT): diagnosis based on 75-g OGTT, 2-hour glucose ≥140 mg/dl (≥7.8 mmol/l) and <200 mg/dl (<11.1 mmol/l)
3. A1C 5.7–6.4%

II. INDICATIONS FOR SCREENING/DIAGNOSTIC TESTING

A. Type 1 diabetes
1. No indications for screening outside of research protocols
2. Diagnostic testing indicated when classic signs and symptoms are present (e.g., polyuria, polydipsia, weight loss, polyphagia, blurred vision)

B. Type 2 diabetes
1. Consider screening at 3-year intervals adults over the age of 45, particularly with a BMI ≥25 kg/m². Screen at a younger age those who are overweight and have one or more of the following risk factors:
   a. Overweight (BMI ≥25* kg/m²) (*may not be correct for all ethnic groups)
   b. Family history of diabetes (parents or siblings or children)
   c. Physically inactive
   d. Race/ethnicity (e.g., Native Americans, African Americans, Latinos, Asian Americans, Pacific Islanders)
   e. Previously identified pre-diabetes (IFG and/or IGT)
   f. History of gestational diabetes or delivery of a baby >9 lb
   g. Hypertension (>140/90 mmHg in adults)
   h. HDL cholesterol <35 mg/dl (0.90 mmol/l) and/or a triglyceride level >250 mg/dl (2.82 mmol/l)
   i. Polycystic ovary syndrome (PCOS)
   j. Acanthosis nigricans
   k. Severe obesity
   l. History of cardiovascular disease (CVD)
2. Screen children and adolescents who are at significant risk for type 2 diabetes. Test every 3 years after the age of 10, or at the onset of puberty if it occurs at a younger age, if:
   a. BMI >85th percentile for age and sex, OR weight for height >85th percentile, OR weight >120% of ideal for height
   b. Family history of type 2 diabetes in first- and second-degree relatives

    c. Belong to certain race/ethnic groups: Native Americans, African Americans, Hispanic Americans, Asians/South Pacific Islanders

    d. Have signs of or conditions associated with insulin resistance (acanthosis nigricans, hypertension, dyslipidemia, PCOS, small for gestational age, birth weight, maternal history of GDM)

C. Gestational diabetes mellitus (GDM)

    1. Risk assessment at first prenatal visit

    2. If high risk, glucose testing as soon as feasible. High risk includes:

        a. Obesity

        b. Previous history of GDM or delivery of large for gestational age baby

        c. Glycosuria

        d. Diabetes in first-degree relative

        e. PCOS

    3. If not high risk, glucose testing is recommended at 24–28 weeks' gestation for all pregnant women except those considered low risk for GDM (see below).

    4. Low-risk status for GDM requires no glucose testing. This status is limited to those women who meet all of the following:

        a. Age <25 years

        b. Normal weight before pregnancy

        c. Member of an ethnic group with a low prevalence of diabetes

        d. No history of abnormal glucose tolerance

        e. No history of poor obstetrical outcomes

    5. One-hour glucose challenge screening test usually between 24 and 28 weeks gestation: plasma glucose (PG) 1 hour after 50-g glucose load:

        a. PG ≥140 mg/dl (7.8 mmol/l) normal screen

        b. PG >140 mg/dl (>7.8 mmol/l) abnormal screen (identifies ~80% of women with GDM)

        c. PG >130 mg/dl (>7.2 mmol/l) abnormal screen (identifies ~90% of women with GDM)

        d. With either abnormal result, diagnostic OGTT indicated; patient undergoes a 100-gram 3-hour OGTT

III. PREPARATION FOR THE OGTT

A. OGTT is performed using a 75-g oral glucose load in the morning after a non-caloric 8-hour fast. Water is allowed.

B. Interfering factors: certain medical conditions, medications, or smoking, exercising, or eating during the test

C. Patients should maintain adequate food intake with adequate carbohyrates (150 g) for at least three days before the test

D. In patients who cannot tolerate oral glucose, IV GT can be performed; values different from OGTT due to rapid absorption with IV GT

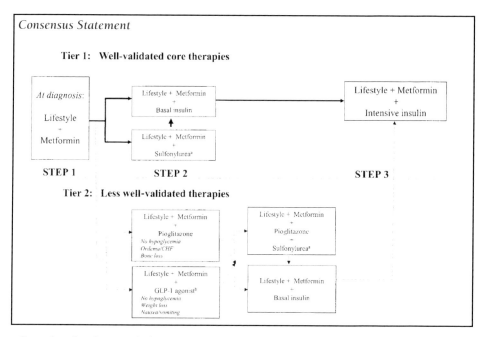

Algorithm for the metabolic management of type 2 diabetes; Reinforce lifestyle interventions at every visit and check A1C every 3 months until A1C <7% and then at least every 6 months. The interventions should be changed if A1C >7%. [a]Sulfonylureas other than glybenclamide (glyburide) or chlorpropamide. [b]Insufficient clinical use to be confident regarding safety. Diabetes Care. *American Diabetes Association, 32 (1), 2009.*

Hospital Admission Guidelines

I. ACUTE METABOLIC COMPLICATIONS OF DIABETES

A. Diabetic ketoacidosis (DKA)
   1. Plasma glucose >250 mg/dl (>13.9 mmol/l) with arterial pH <7.30 and serum bicarbonate level <15 mEq/l and moderate ketonuria and/or ketonemia

B. Hyperosmolar hyperglycemic state (HHS): Impaired mental status and elevated plasma osmolality in a patient with hyperglycemia. Usually includes
   1. Severe hyperglycemia (e.g., plasma glucose >600 mg/dl [>33.3 mmol/l]) and
   2. Elevated serum osmolality (e.g., >320 mOsm/kg [>320 mmol/kg])
   3. pH >7.30
   4. profound dehydration
   5. absence of significant ketoacidosis

C. Severe hypoglycemia with neuroglycopenia
   Blood glucose <50 mg/dl (<2.8 mmol/l) and the treatment of hypoglycemia has not resulted in prompt recovery of sensorium or coma, seizures,

   OR

   altered behavior (e.g., disorientation, ataxia, unstable motor coordination, dysphasia) due to documented or suspected hypoglycemia

II. UNCONTROLLED DIABETES

A. Admission justified when necessary to determine cause and start corrective action. Documentation should include at least one of the following:
   1. Hyperglycemia associated with volume depletion
   2. Persistent refractory hyperglycemia associated with metabolic deterioration
   3. Recurring fasting hyperglycemia >300 mg/dl (>16.7 mmol/l) refractory to outpatient therapy or A1C level 100% above the upper limit of normal
   4. Recurring episodes of severe hypoglycemia (i.e., <50 mg/dl [<2.8 mmol/l]) despite intervention

5. Metabolic instability manifested by frequent swings between hypoglycemia (<50 mg/dl [<2.8 mmol/l]) and fasting hyperglycemia (>300 mg/dl [>16.7 mmol/l])
6. Recurring DKA without precipitating infection or trauma
7. Repeated absence from school or work due to severe psychosocial problems causing poor metabolic control that cannot be managed on an outpatient basis

III. ADDITIONAL FACTORS WARRANTING ADMISSION

A. When there is onset of acute cardiovascular, retinal, renal, or neurological complications of diabetes

B. When presence of diabetes is confounding factor

C. When rapid initiation of rigorous glucose control can improve condition, e.g., pregnancy

D. When primary medical problem or intervention, e.g., large doses of glucocorticoid, can lead to deterioration of glycemic control

Monitoring Glucose Control

I. SELF-MONITORING OF BLOOD GLUCOSE (SMBG)

A. Key element in management of diabetes

B. Glycemic control is best judged by the combination of the results of the patient's SMBG checks and the current A1C result. Continuous glucose monitoring may be appropriate as a supplemental tool to SMBG for certain patients.

C. Patient measures glucose in a blood sample applied to a reagent strip, usually read by a meter. Most meters measure plasma glucose level; older meters read whole blood levels, which are 10–15% lower than plasma levels. Results may be influenced by hematocrit, altitude, temperature, use of oxygen, and other interfering factors (see test strip package).

II. MONITORING IN HOSPITALS REQUIRES:

A. Clear administrative (lab and nursing) responsibility for the procedure

B. Well-defined policy/procedure manual

C. Training program for personnel doing the testing

D. Quality control procedures

E. Regularly scheduled equipment maintenance

III. MONITORING FREQUENCY

A. Determining factors
　　1. Type of diabetes
　　2. Tightness of control preferred (e.g., intensive vs. conventional therapy)
　　3. Ability to perform blood glucose (BG) check independently
　　4. Affordability/reimbursement constraints (e.g., one test strip/day if not requiring insulin)
　　5. Willingness to check BG, e.g., at school, work

B. General guidelines

1. Type 1, insulin pump therapy, pregnancy: three or more times/day, before meals and bedtime and as needed postprandially to optimize therapy, usually postprandial in pregnancy in addition to preprandial

2. Type 2: as needed to achieve glycemic goals and guide therapy: e.g., monitor FPG when adjusting basal insulin or metformin, monitor pre- and post-meals when adjusting mealtime insulin or insulin secretagogues. Continuous glucose monitoring (CGM) in conjunction with intensive insulin regimens can be a useful tool to lower A1C in selected adults (age ≥25 years) with type 1 diabetes and children.

3. GDM: fasting and 1–2 hours after meals

4. Physical activity: generally good idea to check blood glucose 30 minutes before and after to determine risk of hypoglycemia (in type 1 and in type 2, if needed); checks up to 24 hours post-exercise for some people

5. Hypoglycemia: determine presence of hypoglycemia (BG <70 mg/dl) and response to treatment

6. Illness: every 4–6 hours

IV. TARGET PLASMA GLUCOSE LEVELS

Summary of glycemic recommendations for many nonpregnant adults with diabetes

A1C	7.0%
Preprandial capillary plasma glucose	70–130 mg/dl (3.9–7.2 mmol/l)
Peak postprandial capillary plasma glucose	<180 mg/dl (10.0 mmol/l)

A. Goals should be individualized based on:
- duration of diabetes
- age/life expectancy
- comorbid conditions
- known CVD or advanced microvascular complications
- hypoglycemia unawareness
- individual patient considerations

B. More or less stringent glycemic goals may be appropriate for individual patients.

C. Postprandial glucose may be targeted if A1C goals are not met despite reaching preprandial glucose goals. Postprandial glucose measurements should be made

1–2 h after the beginning of the meal, generally peak levels in patients with diabetes. For women with preexisting type 1 or type 2 diabetes who become pregnant, a recent consensus statement recommended the following as optimal glycemic goals, if they can be achieved without excessive hypoglycemia:
1. premeal, bedtime, and overnight glucose 60–99 mg/dl (3.3–5.4 mmol/l)
2. peak postprandial glucose 100–129 mg/dl (5.4 –7.1mmol/l)
3. A1C <6.0%

V. GLYCATED HEMOGLOBIN (A1C)

A. Indicates blood glucose control over a period of several months

B. Normal range varies depending on method lab uses; usually 4–6%, correlating to average blood glucose of ~ 65–136 mg/dl (~5.4–7.1 mmol/l). An A1C range of 5.7–6.4% is used to identify individuals with high risk for future diabetes, a state that may be referred to as prediabetes.

C. Frequency of A1C testing dependent on clinical situation, patient's treatment regimen and clinical judgment.
1. Should be ordered quarterly if not meeting treatment goals and at least twice a year in patients with stable glycemia well within target
2. Availability of A1C result at time of visit has been associated with increased intensification of therapy and improvement in glycemic control

D. Patient does not need to be fasting to have this blood test performed

E. Certain test limitations: e.g., does not provide measure of glycemic variability or hypoglycemia, certain conditions can affect erythrocyte turnover (e.g., hemolysis, blood loss, hemoglobin variants such as sickle cell)

VI. FRUCTOSAMINE TEST (GLYCATED SERUM PROTEIN [GSP])

A. Reflects blood glucose control over preceding 7–10 days; prognostic significance unclear

B. May be used as a means of monitoring women during pregnancy, when more frequent determinations of control are essential, and when hemoglobinopathies exist (fructosamine or glycated albumin can be done instead of A1C for hemoglobinopathies). Each 75 μmol change equals a change of approximately 60 mg/dl blood sugar or 2% HbA1C.

FRUCTOSAMINE TEST LEVELS AND GLUCOSE CONTROL

Test Value	Indication
Under 265 μmol	Normal fructosamine level
265–280	Excellent blood glucose (sugar) control
280–300	Good blood glucose (sugar) control
320–340	Fair blood glucose (sugar) control
Over 350	Poor blood glucose (sugar) control

http://www.isletsofhope.com/diabetes/treatment/tests_fructosamine_1.html Top of Form

VII. URINE/BLOOD KETONE TESTING

A. Ketones
   1. Byproduct of fat metabolism; presence indicates body is not metabolizing food properly due to lack of available insulin or carbohydrate; low ketone levels often seen with fasting, and higher levels together with hyperglycemia may indicate impending or established diabetic ketoacidosis (DKA), a condition that requires immediate medical attention
   2. Should be monitored during severe hyperglycemia or hyperglycemia not responding to therapy in type 1, and pregnancy with preexisting diabetes; may be monitored while fasting or first thing in the morning in GDM

B. Method
   1. Dipstick in urine stream or blood drop applied to ketone (B-hydroxybutyric acid–sensitive) test strip
   2. Blood testing using ketone test strip more accurate and preferred for diagnosing and monitoring ketoacidosis

C. When to test
   1. When blood glucose level is consistently >300 with any type of diabetes, or if patient is sick, stressed, or pregnant, >240 mg/dl in type 1 and not responding to treatment
   2. During periods of acute illness (illness is a stress that can cause hyperglycemia), infection, or stress associated with trauma, injury, or surgery
   3. If pregnant and fasting
   4. When symptoms of hyperglycemia accompanied by nausea, vomiting, abdominal pain, fever, or fruity breath odor are present

Oral Diabetes Medications

I. INDICATIONS: Used as adjunct to meal planning and regular physical activity in type 2 diabetes. Use caution in pregnancy.

II. INSULIN SECRETAGOGUES

Generic Name	Trade Name	Dosage Range	When to Take
A. Sulfonylureas (second generation) long-acting insulin secretagogues			
Glipizide	Glucotrol	5–40 mg	single or divided doses (once daily up to 15, divided up to 40), before meals
Extended Release	Glucotrol XL	5–10 mg	Once daily with meal. Do not chew or crush (20 mg maximum daily dose)
Glyburide	Micronase	1.25–20 mg	1–2 times daily with meals (20 mg maximum daily dose)
	Diabeta	1.25–20 mg	1–2 times daily with meals (20 mg maximum daily dose)
	Glynase	0.75–12 mg	1–2 times daily (12 mg maximum daily dose)
Glimepiride	Amaryl	1–4 mg	Once daily with meal (8 mg maximum daily dose)
B. Short-acting insulin secretagogues			
Meglitinides:			
Repaglinide	Prandin	0.5–4 mg	2–4 times daily within 30 min of meals (16 mg maximum daily dose)
Amino Acid Derivatives:			
Nateglinide	Starlix	60–120 mg	1–3 times daily in equally divided doses (up to 120 mg/meal)

1. Common side effects (not complete list) of sulfonylureas and meglitinides: allergy, hypoglycemia, rash. Risk of hypoglycemia especially in elderly. Pregnancy category C.

III. INSULIN SENSITIZERS

A. Biguanides

Generic Name	Trade Name	Dosage Range	When to Take
Metformin HCl	Glucophage	500–2,550 mg	2–3 divided doses with meals (2,500 mg maximum daily dose)
Metformin	Riomet oral solution	500–2,550 mg	2–3 divided doses with meals (2,550 mg max daily dose)
Metformin HCl Extended	Glucophage XR	500–2,000 mg	1–2 times daily (2,000 mg maximum daily dose)
	Fortamet	500–2,500 mg	Once daily
	Glumetza	500–2,000 mg	Once daily

1. May be used as monotherapy at diagnosis of type 2 diabetes
2. Best taken with meals to minimize GI upset.
3. Common side effects: GI upset, diarrhea, possible resumption of ovulation in premenopausal anovulatory women. When starting, titrate slowly by 500 mg/day at 1-week intervals to minimize GI upset. Confirm normal renal function before starting and monitor (men: creatinine ≤1.5; women: creatinine ≤1.4, especially in elderly). Pregnancy category B.
4. Rare side effect: lactic acidosis if renal, hepatic, or cardiac disease or dysfunction (defined as CHF requiring pharmacologic treatment, acute MI, cardiovascular collapse) is present.
5. Cautions
   a. Due to potential for lactic acidosis with hepatic function impairment, caution patients against excessive alcohol intake, because alcohol potentiates the effect of metformin on lactate metabolism.
   b. Due to potential for lactic acidosis with renal function alteration, temporarily discontinue metformin at the time of or before radiologic studies involving IV Iodinated Contrast Materials. Withhold metformin for 48 hours after procedure and restart medication only after renal function has been reevaluated and determined to be normal.

B. Thiazolidinediones

Rosiglitazone	Avandia**	2–8 mg	1–2 times daily
Pioglitazone	Actos**	15–45 mg	Once daily

**Avandia (rosiglitazone) has been effectively removed from the market because of adverse cardiovascular events. Actos has been removed from the market because of increased risk of bladder cancer.

1. Check liver enzymes before initiating therapy. Do not initiate treatment if ALT >2.5 times the upper normal limits. Liver enzymes should be monitored every 2 months for the first 12 months of therapy and periodically thereafter.
2. Precautions: Symptomatic heart failure. Start at lowest dose and titrate slowly, monitor for edema especially with insulin. Do not use maximum dosing of thiazolidinediones in combination with insulin.
3. Possible resumption of ovulation in premenopausal anovulatory women. Pregnancy category C.
4. Potentiated by CYP2C8 inhibitors (e.g., gemfibrozil), antagonized by CYP2C8 inducers (e.g., rifampin)
5. Risk of fractures and bone loss in women

IV. ALPHA-GLUCOSIDASE INHIBITORS (AGI):

Delay Digestion and Absorption of Carbohydrates in Small Intestine

Acarbose	Precose	25–100 mg ≤ 60kg 150mg/day, ≥ 60kg up to 300 mg/day	1–3 times daily in divided doses at the start of each main meal with first bite
Miglitol	Glyset	25–100 mg	3 times daily at the start of each main meal with first bite (300 mg maximum daily dose)
Linagliptin	Tradjenta	5 mg	Once daily with or without food

1. Common side effects: diarrhea, abdominal discomfort, and flatulence. Walking after meals may reduce flatulence.
2. Not recommended with inflammatory bowel disease, significant renal dysfunction (>2 mg/dl). Monitor serum creatinine and transaminases. Pregnancy category B
3. Must take glucose (not sucrose, etc.) to treat hypoglycemia if taking insulin or insulin secretatogue along with AGI.

V. DPP-IV INHIBITORS

Saxagliptin	2.5 mg or 5 mg	Once daily with or without food
Sitagliptin	100 mg	Once daily with or without food
Linagliptin	5 mg	Once daily with or without food

1. Associated with modest decrease in HbA1C of 0.6%–0.8%; can be dosed with ESRD
2. Minimal side effects (possible more minor infections). There is a risk of hypoglycemia, especially when timing of a sulfonylurea overlaps with action of the DPP-IV inhibitor.

VI. BILE ACID SEQUESTRANTS

A. Colesevelam

Tablets: 1,875 mg (3 tablets) orally twice a day with meals or 3,750 mg (6 tablets) orally once a day with a meal.
Oral suspension: one 3.75 gram packet once daily or one 1.875 gram packet twice daily (mixed with 4 to 8 ounces of water).
1. Add-on therapy for diabetes type 2
2. Side effects may include gas, constipation, nausea, diarrhea, abdominal pain, weakness, muscle pain
3. Initially approved to lower LDL cholesterol; approved for DM2 in 2008
4. Modest efficacy; probably best suited for patients needing small LDL and A1C reductions

VII. COMBINATION ORAL AGENTS

Glyburide/ Metformin HCl	2.5 mg/500 mg to 20 mg/ 2,000 mg (maximum daily dose)	1–2 times daily with meals
Glipizide/ Metformin HC1	2.5 mg/250 mg to 20mg/ 2,000 mg (maximum daily dose)	1–2 times daily with meals
Rosiglitazone/ Metformin HC1	1 mg/500 mg 8 mg/2,000 mg	1–2 times daily with meals
Pioglitazone HCl/ Metformin HCl	15 mg/500 mg 15 mg/850 mg 45 mg/2,550 mg (maximum daily dose adminis- tered in divided doses with food)	1–2 times daily with meals
Pioglitazone HCl/ Metformin HCl XR	15 mg/1000 mg 0 mg/1000 mg 45 mg/2,550 mg (maximum daily dose adminis- tered in divided doses with food)	Once daily with meal
Pioglitazone/ Glimepiride	Starting dose should be based on the patient's current regimen of pioglitazone and/or sulfonylurea 30 mg/2 mg 30 mg/4 mg 45 mg/8 mg maximum daily dose	Once daily
Rosiglitazone maleate/ Glimepiride	4 mg/1 mg (starting dose recommended) 4 mg/2 mg 8 mg/4mg (maximum daily dose)	1–2 times daily with meal
Sitagliptin/ Metformin HCl	50 mg/500 mg 50 mg/1,000 mg (maximum daily dose)	Twice daily with meals
Repaglinide/ Metformin HCl	1 or 2 mg/500 mg 10mg/2,500 mg (maximum daily dose)	2–3 times daily with food

Refer to appropriate drug category for a list of common side effects.

VIII. NON-INSULIN INJECTABLES:

A. Amylin analog(pramlintide): Symlin dosage varies before meals, usually at the same time as insulin injection

B. Incretin GLP-1 analogues: (possible side effects: nausea, vomiting, headache, diarrhea, dizziness)
  1. Exenatide (Byetta) initiate at 5 mcg twice daily within 60 minutes prior to morning and evening meals (or before the two main meals of the day, approximately 6 hours or more apart); increase to 10 mcg twice daily after 1 month based on clinical response. Exenatide carries a higher risk of pancreatitis and pancreatic cancer.
  2. Liraglutide (Victoza) pre-filled, multi-dose pen delivers doses of 0.6 mg, 1.2 mg, or 1.8 mg (6 mg/ml, 3 ml); given once daily at any time of day, independently of meals. Liraglutide carries a higher risk of thyroid tumors.

Insulin and Insulin Therapy

I. INDICATIONS: Always used in patients with type 1 diabetes or DKA and may be required in patients with type 2 or gestational diabetes. For type 1 diabetes, only pramlintide is an approved combination with insulin. Pramlintide also can be used for type 2 diabetes together with insulin.

II. MECHANISM OF ACTION: Facilitates the transport of glucose into cells, promotes glycogen storage, and inhibits fat and protein breakdown.

III. SOURCES

A. Human insulin recombinant, insulin analog: recombinant DNA technology

IV. PREPARATIONS

A. Strength: U-100 (U.S.), U-500 regular insulin is available but rarely used.

B. Type and action

Preparation	Onset (hours)	Duration (hours)
Rapid-acting		
Insulin lispro (analog)	<0.25	3.5–4.5
Insulin aspart (analog)	<0.25	3–5
Insulin glulisine	≤0.25	2–4
Short-acting		
Insulin injection regular (soluble)	0.5	24
Intermediate-acting		
Insulin isophane (NPH) regular	0.5	24
Long-acting		
Insulin detemir	1.0	24
Insulin glargine (analog)	1.1	≥24
Combinations		
70% NPH, 30% regular	0.5	24
70% NPA, 30% aspart	<0.25	24
75% NPL, 25% lispro	≤0.25	24
50% NPL, 50% lispro	≤0.25	16

V. ABSORPTION OF INSULIN

May vary with each patient because of:

A. Source of insulin: human recombinant DNA vs. analog (human insulin tends to have a longer duration of action)

B. Manufacturer: Aventis, Lilly, or Novo Nordisk

C. Injection sites, listed in order of most rapid absorption: abdomen, arm, thigh, buttocks, especially with rapid- and short-acting insulins and combinations

D. Absorption may also be affected by temperature, exercise, lipohypertrophy, massaging injection site.

VI. DOSING

A. Goals
1. Type 1: attempt to mimic body's normal basal/bolus secretion of insulin (physiologic replacement)
2. Type 2: insulin supplementation, progressing to physiologic replacement

B. Examples of individualized insulin regimens:
1. Rapid- or short-acting insulin t.i.d. with meals and intermediate- or long-acting insulin once or twice/day
2. Rapid- or short-acting insulin t.i.d. with meals and intermediate- or long-acting insulin b.i.d.
3. Insulin pump basal rates with premeal and correction boluses
4. Intermediate- or long-acting insulin mixed with rapid- or short-acting insulin b.i.d.
5. Intermediate- or long-acting insulin q.d. or b.i.d. (for type 2 or gestational diabetes)

C. Typical maintenance dose based on weight; starting dose may need to be lower
1. Type 1: 0.5–1.0 units per kg per day
2. Type 2: 0.3–1.5 units per kg per day

VII. TIME OF ADMINISTRATION

A. Will vary depending on type of insulin, e.g., rapid-acting insulin is given within 5–15 minutes of eating; short-acting insulin is given ~30 minutes before meal.

B. May also vary according to blood glucose result, e.g., if premeal glucose is higher than premeal target range, allow time for administered insulin to begin to decrease premeal glucose value before eating.

VIII. EQUIPMENT

A. Syringes (3/10 cc, 1/2 cc, 1 cc; short needles available for children and adults, 1/2 unit markings on some syringes)

B. Insulin pens, pen needles (Use the smallest needles possible to ensure subcutaneous injection and not intradermal or intramuscular.)

C. Insulin pumps

IX. INSULIN ADMINISTRATION GUIDELINES

A. Preparing a single dose
1. Wash hands.
2. If using cloudy insulin, roll vial to mix; do not shake.
3. Draw air into syringe equal to the amount of insulin being withdrawn (equalizes pressure).
4. Insert needle into stopper.
5. Inject air into vial.
6. Invert vial.
7. Fill syringe with insulin.
8. Clear air bubbles.
9. Check dose before administering.

B. Preparing a mixed dose (rare, given shift to premixed vials or pens)
1. Follow steps 1–4 of single dose.
2. Inject air into cloudy insulin first, then remove needle.
3. Draw air into syringe again.
4. Inject air into clear insulin.
5. Invert vial.
6. Fill syringe with clear insulin first.
7. Clear air bubbles.
8. Check dose.
9. Insert needle into cloudy insulin
10. Invert cloudy vial.

11. Fill syringe with cloudy insulin to a combined total of clear and cloudy insulin.
12. Check dose before administering.

C. Injection sites, in order of most rapid to slowest absorption
1. Abdomen has best absorption and is preferred site for mealtime and correction insulin.
2. Upper arm and outer aspect (not deltoid)—difficult for patients to inject in back of arm, may inject muscle and insulin will work too fast
3. Thigh for intermediate- and long-acting insulins
4. Buttocks/flank—very slow absorption, difficult for patients to reach

D. Technique
1. Begin with clean hands and clean injection area. Use of alcohol to prepare site is optional.
2. Pinch injection area skin.
3. Insert needle slowly at 90° angle all the way to hub of syringe.
4. Gradually release pinch as insulin is being injected.
5. Pull needle out at same angle as inserted (do not rub injection site after removal of needle).
6. Insulin syringe may be safely reused a few times; recap needle immediately, and do not wipe needle with alcohol, which removes the silicone coating.
7. U500 insulin is 5 times more concentrated than U100. Care must be taken when measuring dose that every syringe unit measured is understood to be 5 units (regular insulin only).
8. Insulin pumps: Only rapid- and short-acting insulins may be used in insulin pumps.
9. Insulin pens: pen needles come in various sizes (12.7, 8, 6, 5, 4 mm)
10. Refillable and disposable pens, half unit pens, pens with dose memory; premix needs to be mixed every time.

X. INSULIN STORAGE AND DISPOSAL

A. Refrigerate unopened insulin (will be good until the expiration date on the vial).

B. If using vial of insulin within 30 days of opening, may store at room temperature (safety range 37–85°F) or refrigerate (~45°F); most insulin expires after 30 days at room temperature (see package insert).

C. Prefilled syringes (single formulations or approved mixtures) must be kept refrigerated and used within 21 days.

D. Prefilled disposable pens recommendation: keep out of the refrigerator for 28 days after opened.

XI. MIXING INSULINS

A. NPH and short-acting insulin formulations when mixed may be used immediately or stored in refrigerator for up to 2 weeks.

B. Acidity of insulin glargine prevents mixing with another insulin. Do not mix detemir with any other insulin.

C. Educate about responsible disposal of syringes, pen needles, lancets. Local regulations may vary. Check with local waste management authorities.

XII. SIDE EFFECTS OF INSULIN ADMINISTRATION

A. Hypoglycemia

B. Allergic reaction (local/systemic)

C. Lipohypertrophy (thickening of subcutaneous fat at injection site)

D. Lipoatrophy (thinning of subcutaneous fat at injection site)

Medication Effects on Glucose Control

I. DRUGS THAT MAY ALTER GLYCEMIC EFFECT OF SULFONYLUREAS

Drugs that decrease effect of insulin:	Drugs that increase effect of insulin:
Corticosteriods Birth Control Pills/Patches, Estrogens Sympathomimetic Amines Thyroid Hormones Nicotine Clozapine (Clozaril®) Olanzapine (Zyprexa®)	Alcohol Aspirin (large doses) B-Adrenergic Blocker*

May mask signs and symptoms of hypoglycemia

II. DRUGS THAT INTERACT WITH INSULIN EFFECT

A. Increase hypoglycemic effect and decrease blood glucose	B. Decrease hypoglycemic effect and increase blood glucose
ACE inhibitors	Acetazolamide
Alcohol	AIDS antivirals
Anabolic steroids	Albuterol
Antidiabetic products, oral	Asparaginase
β-blockers*	Calcitonin
Calcium	Contraceptives, oral
Chloroquine	Corticosteroids
Clofibrate	Cyclophosphamide
Clonidine	Danazol
Disopyramide	Dextrothyroxine
Fluoxetine	Diazoxide
Guanethidine	Diltiazem
Lithium carbonate	Diuretics
MAO inhibitors	Dobutamine
Mebendazole	Epinephrine
Pentamidine†	Estrogens
Phenylbutazone	Ethacrynic acid
Propoxyphene	Isoniazid
Pyridoxine	Lithium carbonate
Salicylates	Morphine sulfate
Somatostatin analog (e.g., octreotide)	Niacin
Sulfinpyrazone	Nicotine
Sulfonamides	Phenothiazines
Tetracyclines	Phenytoin
	Somatropin
	Terbutaline
	Thiazide diuretics
	Thyroid hormones

*May delay recovery from hypoglycemia or mask signs and symptoms.
† May sometimes be followed by hyperglycemia.

Hypoglycemia/Hyperglycemia

I. HYPOGLYCEMIA (BG <70 MG/DL)

A. Causes
1. Omitted or inadequate food
2. Increased activity
3. Taking too much diabetes medication
4. Erratic or altered absorption of insulin or food
   (e.g., diabetic gastroparesis)

B. Signs and symptoms
1. Mild
   a. Cold, clammy skin; pallor
   b. Weakness/tremors
   c. Excessive hunger
   d. Palpitations
   e. Sweating
2. Moderate
   a. Headache/dizziness
   b. Mood changes/irritability
   c. Drowsiness
   d. Decreased attentiveness
   e. Slurred speech
   f. Slowed reaction time
   g. Blurred vision
3. Severe
   a. Unresponsiveness
   b. Disoriented behavior
   c. Convulsions
   d. Coma

C. Treatment
1. Mild
   a. Give 10–15 g carbohydrate (glucose tabs, 4 oz juice, or regular soda).

  b. Wait 15 minutes, then recheck BG.

  c. If still <70 mg/dl (<3.9 mmol/l) or symptoms remain, repeat treatment.

  d. When ≥70 mg/dl (≥3.9 mmol/l) and symptoms have subsided, if meal or snack not planned within 30 minutes, give extra snack of complex carbohydrate and protein (e.g., cheese and crackers).

2. Moderate: see above; up to 30 g fast-acting carbohydrate (e.g., glucose tablets or gel) may be needed

3. Severe (BG <40 mg/dl, requires assistance from others)

  a. Glucagon SC or IM, dose by age: adult—1mg, children < 5 yrs—0.5mg, infants—0.25mg

    OR

  b. IV dextrose: 12.5–25 g ml administered IV push as 50% glucose slowly over 1–3 minutes; follow with IV glucose solution as ordered by MD/NP/PA. Note: D50 may sometimes precipitate severe neurologic symptoms (Wernicke's encephalopathy) in thiamine deficient patients, e.g., alcoholics. (This can be prevented by administering 100 mg of thiamine IV.)

II. HYPERGLYCEMIA

A. Diabetic ketoacidosis (DKA). More commonly seen with type 1 diabetes but some ketosis may occur with type 2 diabetes.

 1. Causes

  a. Illness—urinary tract infection or pneumonia are most common causes

  b. Omission of insulin

  c. Sick-day mismanagement

 2. Symptoms and signs

  a. Diagnostic criteria:

   • Elevated glucose level (>250 mg/dl [>13.9 mmol/l]) and ketones

   • Arterial pH <7.30

   • Serum bicarbonate <18 mEq/l

   • Anion gap >10

   • Ketonuria and/or ketonemia

  b. Other presenting factors:

   • Increased thirst and urination

   • Abdominal pain

- Nausea and vomiting
- Dehydration
- Hyperpnea or Kussmaul breathing; acetone odor
- Weakness and/or anorexia
- Warm, dry skin; tachycardia; flushed face

3. **Prevention:** Check ketones if glucose is >240 mg/dl (>13.3 mmol/l).
4. **Treatment**
   a. Requires hospitalization to correct life-threatening abnormalities
   b. Approaches to management in adults and pediatric patients provided on following pages
   c. IV fluids
      - Potassium replacement
      - IV insulin

B. **Hyperosmolar hyperglycemic state (HHS)**
   1. Causes
      a. Therapeutic agents such as thiazides, propranolol, phenytoin, steroids, furosemide, and chlorthalidone may precipitate the onset of HHS
      b. Chronic disease-concomitant illnesses such as pneumonia, acute myocardial infarction, pancreatitis, etc. More common among elderly with type 2 diabetes, often institutionalized in long-term care settings.
      c. Acute infection
      d. Thirst disturbance or inability to access water (dementia, bedridden patient)
   2. Symptoms and signs: same as DKA, with the following exceptions:
      a. Prolonged hyperglycemia: >600 mg/dl (>33.3 mmol/l), often 1000–2000 mg/dl [55.5–111.0 mmol/l]
      b. Severe dehydration
      c. Absence of or slight ketosis
      d. Plasma or serum hyperosmolality (>320 mOsm/kg), serum K normal, Na may be low or high, arterial pH often >7.3
      e. Confusion/coma; altered mental status
      f. Usually no nausea, vomiting, or abdominal pain
   3. Treatment
      a. Requires immediate hospitalization to correct life-threatening abnormalities
      b. Approach to management in adults and pediatric patients provided on the following pages; treatment: IV saline and insulin

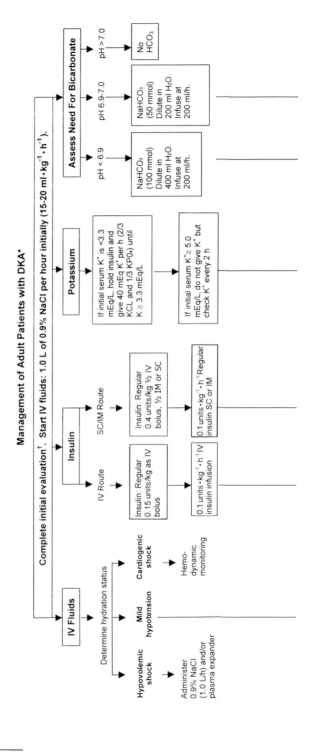

Management of Adult Patients with DKA*

Complete initial evaluation†. Start IV fluids: 1.0 L of 0.9% NaCl per hour initially (15-20 ml·kg⁻¹·h⁻¹).

IV Fluids

Determine hydration status

- **Hypovolemic shock**
  - Administer 0.9% NaCl (1.0 L/h) and/or plasma expander
- **Mild hypotension**
- **Cardiogenic shock**
  - Hemo-dynamic monitoring

Insulin

- **IV Route**
  - Insulin: Regular 0.15 units/kg as IV bolus
  - 0.1 units·kg⁻¹·h⁻¹ IV insulin infusion
- **SC/IM Route**
  - Insulin: Regular 0.4 units/kg ½ IV bolus, ½ IM or SC
  - 0.1 units·kg⁻¹·h⁻¹ Regular insulin SC or IM

Potassium

- If initial serum K⁺ is <3.3 mEq/L, hold insulin and give 40 mEq K⁺ per h (2/3 KCL and 1/3 KPO₄) until K ≥ 3.3 mEq/L
- If initial serum K⁺≥ 5.0 mEq/L, do not give K⁺ but check K⁺ every 2 h

Assess Need For Bicarbonate

- **pH < 6.9**
  - NaHCO₃ (100 mmol) Dilute in 400 ml H₂O. Infuse at 200 ml/h.
- **pH 6.9-7.0**
  - NaHCO₃ (50 mmol) Dilute in 200 ml H₂O. Infuse at 200 ml/h.
- **pH >7.0**
  - No HCO₃

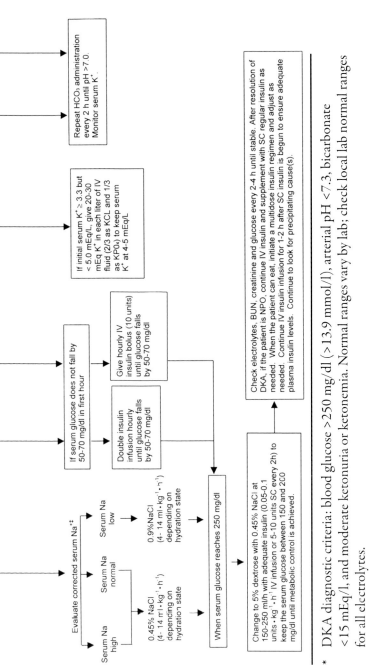

Repeat HCO₃ administration every 2 h until pH >7.0. Monitor serum K⁺.

If initial serum K⁺ ≥ 3.3 but < 5.0 mEq/L, give 20-30 mEq K⁺ in each liter of IV fluid (2/3 as KCL and 1/3 as KPO₄) to keep serum K⁺ at 4-5 mEq/L

Give hourly IV insulin bolus (10 units) until glucose falls by 50-70 mg/dl

If serum glucose does not fall by 50-70 mg/dl in first hour

Double insulin infusion hourly until glucose falls by 50-70 mg/dl

Evaluate corrected serum Na⁺‡

Serum Na high | Serum Na normal | Serum Na low

0.45% NaCl (4 - 14 ml·kg⁻¹·h⁻¹) depending on hydration state

0.9%NaCl (4 - 14 ml·kg⁻¹·h⁻¹) depending on hydration state

When serum glucose reaches 250 mg/dl

Change to 5% dextrose with 0.45% NaCl at 150-250 ml/h with adequate insulin (0.05-0.1 units·kg⁻¹·h⁻¹ IV infusion or 5-10 units SC every 2h) to keep the serum glucose between 150 and 200 mg/dl until metabolic control is achieved.

Check electrolytes, BUN, creatinine and glucose every 2-4 h until stable. After resolution of DKA, if the patient is NPO, continue IV insulin and supplement with SC regular insulin as needed. When the patient can eat, initiate a multidose insulin regimen and adjust as needed. Continue IV insulin infusion for 1-2 h after SC insulin is begun to ensure adequate plasma insulin levels. Continue to look for precipitating cause(s).

* DKA diagnostic criteria: blood glucose >250 mg/dl (>13.9 mmol/l), arterial pH <7.3, bicarbonate <15 mEq/l, and moderate ketonuria or ketonemia. Normal ranges vary by lab; check local lab normal ranges for all electrolytes.

† After history and physical examination, obtain arterial blood gases, complete blood count with differential, urinalysis, blood glucose, blood urea nitrodgen (BUN), electrolytes, chemistry profile, and creatinine levels STAT as well as an electrocardiogram. Obtain chest X-ray and cultures as needed.

‡ Serum Na should be corrected for hyperglycemia: for each 100 mg/dl glucose >100 mg/dl, add 1.6 mEq to sodium value for corrected serum sodium.

Management of Pediatric Patients (<20 years) with DKA* or HHS†

Complete initial evaluation‡. Start IV fluids: 10-20 ml/kg, 0.9% NaCl in the initial hour.

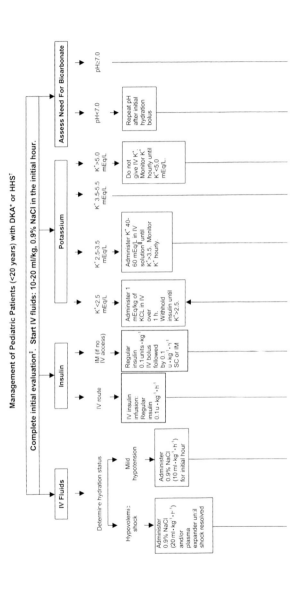

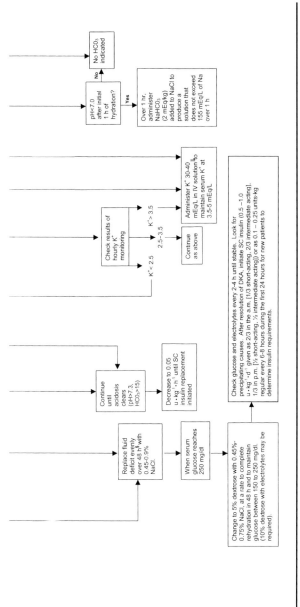

No HCO₃ indicated → No HCO₃ indicated

pH<7.0 after initial 1 h of hydration?

No

No HCO₃ indicated

Yes

Over 1 hr, administer NaHCO₃ (2 mEq/kg) added to NaCl to produce a solution that does not exceed 155 mEq/L of Na over 1 h

Check results of hourly K⁺ monitoring

K⁺ < 2.5

2.5–3.5

K⁺ > 3.5

Administer K⁺ 30–40 mEq/L in IV solution‖ to maintain serum K⁺ at 3.5-5 mEq/L

Continue as above

Continue until acidosis clears (pH>7.3, HCO₃>15)

Decrease to 0.05 u · kg⁻¹ · h⁻¹ until SC insulin replacement initiated

Replace fluid deficit evenly over 48 h# with 0.45–0.9% NaCl.

When serum glucose reaches 250 mg/dl

Change to 5% dextrose with 0.45%-0.75% NaCl, at a rate to complete rehydration in 48 h and to maintain glucose between 150 to 250 mg/dl. (10% dextrose with electrolytes may be required).

Check glucose and electrolytes every 2-4 h until stable. Look for precipitating causes. After resolution of DKA, initiate SC insulin (0.5 –1.0 u · kg⁻¹ · d⁻¹ given as 2/3 in the a.m. [1/3 short-acting, 2/3 intermediate acting], 1/3 in p.m. [½ short-acting, ½ intermediate acting]) or as 0.1 – 0.25 units·kg regular every 6-8 hours during the first 24 hours for new patients to determine insulin requirements.

---

* KA diagnostic criteria: blood glucose >250 mg/dl (>13.9 mmol/l), venous pH <7.3, bicarbonate <15 mEq/l, moderate ketonuria or ketonemia.

† HHS diagnostic criteria: blood glucose >600 mg/dl (>33.3 mmol/l), venous pH >7.3, bicarbonate >15 mEq/l, and altered mental status or severe dehydration.

‡ After history and physical examination, obtain blood glucose, venous blood gases, electrolytes, blood urea nitrogen (BUN), creatinine, calcium, phosphorous, and urine analysis STAT.

§ Usually 1.5 times the 24-h maintenance requirements (~5 ml) will accomplish a smooth rehydration; do not exceed two times the maintenance requirement.

‖ The potassium in solution should be 1/3 KPO₄ and 2/3 KCl or Kacetate.

Management of Adult Patients with HHS*

Complete initial evaluation†. Start IV fluids: 1.0 L of 0.9% NaCl per hour initially.

```
        ┌──────────┐         ┌──────────┐         ┌──────────┐
        │ IV Fluids │         │ Insulin  │         │Potassium │
        └──────────┘         └──────────┘         └──────────┘
```

IV Fluids

Determine hydration status

Hypovolemic shock → Administer 0.9% NaCl (1.0 L/h) and/or plasma expanders

Cardiogenic shock → Hemodynamic monitoring

Mild hypotension

Insulin

Regular, 0.15 units/kg as IV bolus

0.1 units · kg⁻¹ · h⁻¹ IV insulin infusion

Potassium

If initial serum K⁺ is <3.3 mEq/L, hold insulin and give 40 mEq K⁺ (2/3 as KCl and 1/3 KPO₄) until K⁺ ≥ 3.3 mEq/L

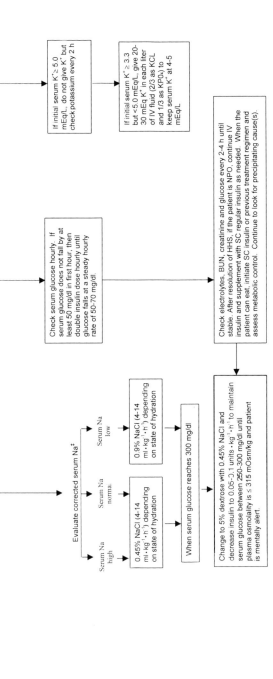

If initial serum K⁺ ≥ 5.0 mEq/L, do not give K⁺ but check potassium every 2 h

If initial serum K⁺ ≥ 3.3 but <5.0 mEq/L, give 20-30 mEq K⁺ in each liter of IV fluid (2/3 as KCL and 1/3 as KPO₄) to keep serum K⁺ at 4-5 mEq/L

Check serum glucose hourly. If serum glucose does not fall by at least 50 mg/dl in first hour, then double insulin dose hourly until glucose falls at a steady hourly rate of 50-70 mg/dl.

Check electrolytes, BUN, creatinine and glucose every 2-4 h until stable. After resolution of HHS, if the patient is NPO, continue IV insulin and supplement with SC regular insulin as needed. When the patient can eat, initiate SC insulin or previous treatment regimen and assess metabolic control. Continue to look for precipitating cause(s).

Evaluate corrected serum Na‡

Serum Na high

0.45% NaCl (4-14 ml · kg⁻¹ · h⁻¹) depending on state of hydration

Serum Na normal

0.45% NaCl (4-14 ml · kg⁻¹ · h⁻¹) depending on state of hydration

Serum Na low

0.9% NaCl (4-14 ml · kg⁻¹ · h⁻¹) depending on state of hydration

When serum glucose reaches 300 mg/dl

Change to 5% dextrose with 0.45% NaCl and decrease insulin to 0.05-0.1 units · kg⁻¹ · h⁻¹ to maintain serum glucose between 250-300 mg/dl until plasma osmolality is ≤ 315 mOsm/kg and patient is mentally alert.

---

* Diagnostic criteria: blood glucose >600 mg/dl (>33.3 mmol/l), arterial pH >7.3, bicarbonate >15 mEq/l, mild ketonuria or ketonemia, and effective serum osmalality >320 mOsm/kg H₂O. This protocol is for patients admitted with mental status change or severe dehydration who require admission to an intensive care unit. For less severe cases, see text for management guidelines. Normal ranges vary by lab; check local lab normal ranges for all electrolytes. Effective serum osmolality calculation: 2/measured Na (mEq/l) + glucose (mg/dl)/18.

† After history and physical examination, obtain arterial blood gases, complete blood count with differential, urinalysis, plasma glucose, blood urea nitrodgen (BUN), electrolytes, chemistry profile, and creatinine levels STAT as well as an electrocardiogram. Obtain chest X-ray and cultures as needed.

‡ Serum Na should be corrected for hyperglycemia: for each 100 mg/dl glucose >100 mg/dl, add 1.6 mEq to sodium value for corrected serum value.

Chronic Complications of Diabetes

I. ACCELERATED MACROVASCULAR DISEASE

Cardiovascular disease is the leading cause of morbidity and mortality among people with diabetes. Type 2 diabetes is an independent risk factor for cardiovascular disease.

A. **Additional risk factors**
1. Hypertension
2. Dyslipidemia
3. Smoking
4. Family history of heart disease at an early age (<55 years in male and <65 years in female first-degree relatives)
5. Obesity

B. **Common manifestations**
1. Angina, classic symptoms: chest, arm, and/or jaw pain (discomfort); shortness of breath; cold, clammy sweat
2. Myocardial infarction (MI): "silent" MI more common in diabetes population; may be unusual or no symptoms with either angina or MI in diabetes. Sometimes presents as abdominal pain, fatigue, and dizziness. Symptoms are often not experienced because of autonomic neuropathy.
3. Dyslipidemia: treated more aggressively than in general population; goals are
   a. LDL <100 mg/dl (<2.6 mmol/l), high risk patients with overt CVD <70 mg/dl
   b. HDL >40 mg/dl (>1.1 mmol/l) for men, >50 mg/dl (>1.4 mmol/l) for women
   c. Triglycerides <150 mg/dl (<1.7 mmol/l); A1C <7%
4. Hypertension: goal in diabetes is <130/80 mmHg
5. Peripheral vascular disease
6. Cerebral vascular disease

II. MICROVASCULAR DISEASE

A. **Retinopathy:** leading cause of new cases of blindness in adults
1. Progression
   a. Nonproliferative retinopathy: microaneurysms and hard matter (exudates) found with ophthalmoscopic exam

b. Proliferative retinopathy: formation of new, fragile blood vessels to replace less functional capillaries in the retinal circulation; development carries substantial risk of severe hemorrhage and retinal detachment

c. Macular edema, tractional retinal detachment, and neovascular glaucoma associated with proliferative retinopathy are common causes of vision loss.

2. Blindness prevention

a. Those age ≥10 years (type 1) within 5 yrs of diagnosis need an annual dilated and comprehensive eye exam by eye care professional, Those with type 2 need an eye exam at diagnosis and annually

b. Optimize hypertension, blood glucose, and dyslipidemia control

c. Any level of macular edema or nonproliferative or proliferative retinopathy requires referral to ophthalmologist for possible treatment, including laser photocoagulation

B. **Nephropathy:** most common single cause of end-stage renal disease

1. Progression

a. Characterized by hypertension, edema, proteinuria, and renal insufficiency

b. Development of end-stage renal disease may require dialysis or renal transplant

2. Prevention

a. Optimize hypertension and blood glucose control

b. Albuminuria testing identifies early kidney disease, based on spot collection:

Category	Spot collection (g/mg creatinine)
Normal	<30
Microalbuminuria	30–299 (slow progression with possible damage)
Macro (clinical)—albuminuria	≥300 (overt diabetic nephropathy)

C. Neuropathy: can affect virtually any body part, but neuropathic loss of sensation in the foot commonly conspires with infection and/or vascular insufficiency to produce the most frequent cause of nontraumatic lower-limb amputation

1. Peripheral
   a. Diabetic Peripheral Neuropathy (DPN): most common, usually progressive
      - Unsteadiness, ataxic gait, and weakness in muscles of hands and feet; result of diminished proprioception (diminished sense of body position) and light touch
      - Diminished pain and temperature sensation
      - Typical touch sensation may become uncomfortable and progress to loss of sensation
      - Distal to proximal (stocking-glove) pattern of distribution typical
      - Extreme hypersensitivity to light touch, superficial burning, stabbing pain, bone-deep aching or tearing pain, usually most troublesome at night
      - Foot ulcerations, infections, and neuroarthropathy (Charcot's joint—joint erosion, unrecognized fractures, bone demineralization); risk can be reduced with proper foot care
      - Sometimes asymptomatic; if symptoms occur, may be self-limiting or progressive
   b. Focal neuropathies: sudden onset, usually improve over time
      - Cranial: third nerve—presenting with unilateral pain, diplopia, and ptosis
      - Radiculopathy: nerve roots—presents as band-like thoracic or abdominal or truncal pain
      - Plexopathy: brachial or lumbosacral plexus—pain that radiates to extremities
2. Autonomic
   a. Orthostatic hypotension
   b. Cardiac denervation syndrome; interferes with cardiovascular reflexes
      - Heart hypersensitive to circulating catecholamines
      - Dysrhythmias, most often tachycardia
      - Altered exercise tolerance
      - Silent MI (painless)
      - Sudden death

c. Gastrointestinal neuropathy (gastroparesis)
- Delayed gastric emptying (nausea and vomiting with gastroparesis)
- Decreased motility
- Delayed nutrient absorption
- Constipation/diarrhea

d. Genitourinary neuropathy
- Erectile dysfunction
- Retrograde ejaculation with potential infertility
- Arousal disorder and/or painful intercourse
- Bladder dysfunction

e. Hypoglycemia unawareness: blunted response of counterregulatory hormones (epinephrine, glucagon, cortisol, growth hormone) to hypoglycemia

f. Autonomic sudomotor dysfunction
- Uncontrolled anhidrosis of extremities
- Gustatory sweating (central hyperhidrosis)
- Prevention
- Prompt and proper diagnosis
- Optimize blood glucose control

Illness

I. DEFINITION

A. Illness is a stress that can lead to poor glucose control in both type 1 and type 2 diabetes. It aggravates glycemic control by increasing counterregulatory hormones and cytokines and frequently leads to ketoacidosis in type 1 diabetes, necessitating more frequent monitoring of blood glucose and urine or blood ketones, and additional insulin.

B. Nausea and vomiting accompanied by ketosis may indicate diabetic ketoacidosis (DKA), a life-threatening condition that requires immediate medical care to prevent complications and death; the possibility of DKA should always be considered.

C. Infection or dehydration is more likely to necessitate hospitalization of the person with diabetes. Aggressive glycemic management with IV insulin and fluids may reduce morbidity in patients with severe acute illness.

II. MEDICATION

A. Changes in diabetes medication are usually necessary during the physical stress of illness or surgery.

B. Patients must continue to take routine insulin (even if vomiting and unable to eat) or oral diabetes medication, as illness is likely to raise blood glucose.

C. Patients taking insulin may require correction regular or rapid-acting insulin every 3–4 hours based on glucose results and advice of health care provider.

D. Patients treated with oral diabetes medication or lifestyle changes alone may need to switch to insulin temporarily or to change dose, based on blood glucose results and advice from health care provider.

III. MONITORING

A. Blood glucose monitoring is required to guide adjustments and maintain adequate glycemic control.

B. Blood glucose should be tested at least every 2–4 hours; Blood glucose levels should be checked by the laboratory if they exceed the linearity range of the meter.

C. Urine and blood ketones: if glucose >240 mg/dl (>13.3 mmol/l), urine or blood should be tested for ketones every 3–4 hours; patient should report moderate to large ketone levels to health care provider.

IV. SICK-DAY NUTRITION GUIDELINES (INPATIENT OR OUTPATIENT)

A. Nutrition needs vary based on type of illness, diagnostic procedure, or surgery. Regardless of the type of feeding used (e.g., consistent carbohydrate meal plan, clear liquids, enteral or parenteral feedings), adequate fluid and caloric intake is essential.

B. Nutritional recommendations should be individualized based on treatment goals, physiologic parameters, and medication usage.

  1. Fluid replacement

    a. To prevent dehydration, which may be related to fever, diarrhea, nausea, and vomiting, at least 4–8 oz water or other noncaloric fluids (sugar-free drinks such as broth, tea, water, diet soda) should be consumed hourly. Broth is good for replacement of salt lost with dehydration.

    b. For nausea and vomiting, small sips of fluids or ice chips should be taken every 15–20 minutes. An antiemetic is often required.

    c. When a consistent carbohydrate meal cannot be consumed, carbohydrate (CHO) in the meal should be replaced with fluids or soft foods. Examples of fluids containing 10–15 g CHO:

- 1/2 cup regular soft drink
- 1 cup Gatorade
- 1/2 cup fruit juice
- 1 cup of soup (with noodles or rice)

    d. Enteral feedings

- For tube feedings, a standard enteral formula (50% CHO) or a lower-carbohydrate enteral formula (33–40% CHO) may be used.

    e. Total parenteral nutrition (TPN)

- TPN is a form of IV nutrition used when a long-term alternative is needed for those unable to be fed orally or by tube.
- Standard and customized solutions are available for both central and peripheral IV access. Base formula includes a prescribed percentage of amino acids, dextrose, and fat established for the

patient's needs. Electrolyte components are added to the solution in standard or customized amounts.

- Insulin is added to the solution based on blood glucose levels. Blood glucose monitoring and lab protocols should be based on the patient's condition.

2. Meal replacement

   a. When patient is again able to consume food, small, frequent meals containing 10–15 g CHO can be taken every 1–2 hours while awake.

   b. Examples of food containing 10–15 g carbohydrate:
      - 1/2 cup sweetened gelatin
      - 1 slice toast or bread
      - 1 regular double Popsicle
      - 3 graham crackers
      - 6 saltine crackers
      - 1/4 cup sherbet
      - 1/2 cup custard or pudding
      - 6 vanilla wafers
      - 1/2 cup ice cream
      - 1/2 cup cooked cereal
      - 1/2 cup mashed potatoes

V. INFORMATION NEEDED FROM PATIENT WHEN ILL

A. Length of illness

B. Glucose and urine or blood ketone levels

C. Presence and duration of diarrhea, nausea, or vomiting (if >4 hours)

D. Change in body weight since onset of illness

E. Any other symptoms (e.g., abdominal pain, shortness of breath)

F. Fever (if >101°F)

G. Medications: dose, times of insulin injections, injection sites, and other medications taken

H. Quantity and kinds of food and fluids consumed during day

Management of Glycemia During Hospitalization and Surgery

I. HOSPITALIZATION

A. Diabetes increases the risk for comorbidities that often result in hospitalization, including coronary artery, cerebrovascular, and peripheral arterial disease; nephropathy; infection; and lower-extremity amputations, but management of diabetes too often becomes secondary to the condition that prompted the admission.

1. Aggressive glycemic management with insulin may reduce morbidity in patients with severe acute illness, perioperatively, and following myocardial infarction. Insulin infusion is safe and effective for achieving metabolic control during major surgery, hemodynamic instability, and NPO status.

2. Blood glucose goals during hospitalization

   a. *Critical care:* Recommended 140–180 mg/dl, Acceptable: 110–140 mg/dl in select patients.

   b. *Non-critical Care*: Random less than 180 mg/dl, premeal <140 mg/dl

3. Use of scheduled basal and meal insulin improves glycemic control compared with orders based on sliding-scale insulin coverage alone.

4. Type 1 patients must receive basal insulin at all times despite reductions or absence of calorie intake and perioperatively to prevent diabetic ketoacidosis.

5. Oral diabetes medications should be discontinued during hospitalization and may be resumed if patient is stable close to or after discharge. An A1C should be done to determine glycemic control prior to admission to assess home therapy.

B. Acute hyperglycemia in the hospital or outpatient/clinic setting

1. May contribute to microvascular and macrovascular complications, prolong length of stays, and contribute to increased morbidity and mortality rates

2. Hyperglycemia and relative insulin deficiency caused by metabolic stress triggers tissue and organ injury via the combined effects of infection, direct fuel-mediated injury, and oxidative stress. Moderate to severe hyperglycemia (mean glucose >200 mg/dl [>11.1 mmol/l]) has been shown to cause or be related to:

a. Immunosuppression (leukocyte dysfunction and reduced T-cell populations)

b. Cellular injury/apoptosis

c. Inflammation

d. Tissue damage

e. Altered tissue/wound repair

f. Acidosis

g. Infarction/ischemia

3. Patients with no prior history of diabetes found to have hyperglycemia (random blood glucose >125 mg/dl [>6.9 mmol/l]) should have an A1C. A1C >6.5% is diagnostic, A1C 5.7–6.4% should indicates high risk and requires outpatient followup.

II. SURGERY

A. Management of diabetes patients requiring surgery focuses on risk reduction by normalizing blood glucose levels during and after surgery. Perioperative hyperglycemia delays healing and increases risk of ischemia.

1. Perioperative plasma glucose levels 80–110 mg/dl (4.5–6.1 mmol/l) reduce morbidity and mortality among critically ill patients in the surgical ICU. Adjust IV insulin and glucose for the individual's insulin requirement titrated from frequent blood glucose values.

2. Customary basal insulin dose is the minimum required to counteract insulin resistance and glucogenesis caused by stress. Additional insulin also will be needed to prevent excessive hepatic glucose release and decreased peripheral utilization while maintaining normal glucose levels and fluid and electrolyte balance.

B. Preoperative planning and assessment

1. Glycemic control and therapy adjusted as appropriate for current therapy and type of surgery

2. Additional assessments if needed, e.g., chest X ray, ECG, renal function, A1C

3. Anesthesia consultation

a. Type 2 treated with lifestyle changes alone

- Assess for metabolic control (A1C)
- Stabilize metabolic control with consistent carbohydrate meal planning and, if necessary, institute insulin therapy, similar to insulin-treated diabetes
- Schedule for surgery in morning

    b. Type 2 treated with oral agents
- Assess for metabolic control (A1C)
- If on long-acting sulfonylurea, change to shorter-acting sulfonylurea 1 week before surgery; may require insulin for stabilization. Discontinue oral agents during hospitalization and order insulin therapy
- Frequent blood glucose monitoring
- If control poor, stop oral agents and start insulin therapy

    c. Type 1 or type 2 treated with insulin
- May require admission 1 day before major surgery for assessment and possible stabilization of glycemic control

C. Minor, elective surgery
1. Patients undergoing elective surgery with local anesthesia (e.g., dental work) should eat only after surgery.
2. Patients treated with lifestyle changes only or oral agents who are in good metabolic control usually don't require insulin.
3. Withhold food and short-acting insulin and continue basal insulin as insulin glargine or via insulin pump. If patient is managed in some other manner, they should be switched to a basal-bolus program before an elective procedure.
4. Monitor blood glucose 1–2 times/hour initially, reducing frequency as appropriate.
5. Place on IV insulin and glucose several hours preoperatively and maintain at <180 mg/dl (5.5–8.3 mmol/l).

D. Emergency surgery requiring general anesthesia: there is usually sufficient time to optimally evaluate and stabilize the patient. DKA can be treated concurrently with surgery.

E. Intravenous infusion of insulin rather than subcutaneous insulin administration is indicated to allow careful control of the amount and speed of insulin delivery and circumvent problems with subcutaneous absorption in the event of shock. One approach is provided on following pages. Follow your hospital's protocol for intravenous insulin.
1. Four to 8 hours before surgery, keep patient NPO, omit usual SC insulin, and insert IV line. Start infusion of 6.25 g/hour glucose (125 ml/hour D5 0.45% normal saline [NS] with 20 mEq KCl/l). Administer insulin as follows:

a. Deliver 50 units regular insulin in 500 ml NS controlled with an IV regulator pump.

b. Piggyback insulin line into the D5 0.45% NS line.

c. Deliver at a rate (unit/hour) equal to (blood glucose [BG] mg/dl – 60) × 0.02 (or [BG mmol/l – 3.3] × 0.02), where 0.02 is the sensitivity factor (SF).

d. Monitor BG hourly and adjust rate per formula.

e. If BG is not decreasing or increases to >150 mg/dl (>8.3 mmol/l), increase SF by 0.01.

f. If BG is <100 mg/dl (<5.5 mmol/l), decrease SF by 0.01.

g. If BG is <80 mg/dl (<4.4 mmol/l), give IV D50W equal to (100–BG mg/dl) × 0.3 ml or (5.5–BG mmol/l) × 0.3 ml.

h. Continue IV insulin as per formula with new SF.

i. Repeat BG in 30 minutes.

2. After surgery

a. Continue IV insulin and glucose (D5 0.45% NS) infusion until 2 hours after oral feeding is resumed. If patient is NPO for several days, infuse sufficient glucose (150 g/day in adults; 2–4 g/kg/day in children) to meet minimal catabolic needs. Adjust the insulin infusion as per above to maintain BG 100–150 mg/dl (5.5–8.3 mmol/l).

b. Transition to basal insulin such as glargine plus preprandial rapid-acting insulin when patient is able to eat.

c. Long-acting insulin should be given in a dose equal to the average rate per hour of IV insulin infusion over the past 2–6 h × 12, e.g., (120–60) × 0.03 × 12 = 22 units if the last multiplier was 0.03 and the average BG was 120 mg/dl.

d. Rapid-acting insulin should be given after the patient has eaten and in proportion to amount eaten at 1 unit per 10 g carbohydrate.

e. Monitor BG at each meal, bedtime, and 3:00 a.m. Correction doses of rapid-acting insulin should be given for any BG >150 mg/dl (>8.3 mmol/l), per the formula Correction dose (units) = (BG mg/dl – 100)/correction. Correction factor = 1700/daily insulin.

f. For insulin pump patients: resume basal rate and give boluses as per carbohydrate intake plus correction formula as above or according to the patient's existing correction factor.

Diabetes Self-Management Education (DSME)

I. DEFINITION

A. DSME is the cornerstone of care for all individuals with diabetes who want to achieve successful health-related outcomes.

B. The National Standards for DSME are designed to define quality diabetes self-management education that can be implemented in diverse settings and will facilitate improvement in health care outcomes.

II. NATIONAL STANDARDS FOR DSME

Standard 1: The DSME entity will have documentation of its organizational structure, mission statement, and goals and will recognize and support quality DSME as an integral component of diabetes care.

Standard 2: The DSME entity shall appoint an advisory group to promote quality. This group shall include representatives from the health professions, people with diabetes, the community, and other stakeholders.

Standard 3: The DSME entity will determine the diabetes educational needs of the target population(s) and identify resources necessary to meet these needs.

Standard 4: A coordinator will be designated to oversee the planning, implementation, and evaluation of diabetes self-management education. The coordinator will have academic or experiential preparation in chronic disease care and education and in program management.

Standard 5: DSME will be provided by one or more instructors. The instructors will have recent educational and experiential preparation in education and diabetes management or will be a certified diabetes educator. The instructor(s) will obtain regular continuing education in the field of diabetes management and education. At least one of the instructors will be a registered nurse, dietitian, or pharmacist. A mechanism must be in place to ensure that the participant's needs are met if those needs are outside the instructors' scope of practice and expertise.

Standard 6: A written curriculum reflecting current evidence and practice guidelines, with criteria for evaluating outcomes, will serve as the framework for the DSME entity. Assessed needs of the individual with pre-diabetes and diabetes will determine which of the content areas listed below are to be provided:

- Describing the diabetes disease process and treatment options
- Incorporating nutritional management into lifestyle
- Incorporating physical activity into lifestyle
- Using medication(s) safely and for maximum therapeutic effectiveness
- Monitoring blood glucose and other parameters and interpreting and using the results for self-management decision making
- Preventing, detecting, and treating acute complications
- Preventing detecting, and treating chronic complications
- Developing personal strategies to address psychosocial issues/concerns
- Developing personal strategies to promote health and behavior change

Standard 7: An individual assessment and education plan will be developed collaboratively by the participant and instructor(s) to direct the selection of appropriate educational interventions and self-management support strategies. This assessment and education plan and the intervention and outcomes will be documented in the education record.

Standard 8: A personalized follow-up plan for ongoing self-management support will be developed collaboratively by the participant and instructor(s). The patient's outcomes and goals and the plan for ongoing self-management support will be communicated to the referring provider.

Standard 9: The DSME entity will measure attainment of patient-defined goals and patient outcomes at regular intervals using appropriate measurement techniques to evaluate the effectiveness of the educational intervention.

Standard 10: The DSME entity will measure the effectiveness of the education process and determine opportunities for improvement using a written continuous quality improvement plan that describes and documents a systematic review of the entities' process and outcome data.

III. OUTCOMES MEASUREMENT OF DSME

A. The primary purposes of DSME are to provide knowledge and skill training, help individuals identify barriers, and facilitate problem solving and coping skills to achieve effective self-care behavior and behavior change.

B. DSME Outcome Standards
1. Behavior change is the unique outcome measurement for DSME.
2. The AADE7 self-care behaviors provide a useful framework for assessment and documentation.
   a. Physical activity
   b. Healthy eating
   c. Medication taking
   d. Monitoring of blood glucose
   e. Diabetes self-care problem solving
   f. Reducing risks of diabetes complications
   g. Living with and coping with diabetes (psychosocial adaptation)
3. Diabetes self-care behaviors should be evaluated at baseline and then at regular intervals during and after the education program.
4. The continuum of outcomes, including learning, behavioral, clinical, and health status, should be assessed to demonstrate the interrelationship between DSME and behavior change in the care of individuals with diabetes.
5. Individual patient outcomes are used to guide the intervention and improve the care for that patient. Aggregate patient outcomes are used to guide programmatic services and for continuous quality improvement activities for DSME and for the population served.

Medical Nutrition Therapy (MNT)

I. DEFINITION

A. People with diabetes should receive individualized MNT as needed over the life span to achieve treatment goals, preferably provided by a registered dietitian familiar with the components of diabetes MNT. This is usually best provided in an outpatient or home care setting.

B. MNT involves a nutrition assessment to evaluate the patient's food intake, metabolic status, lifestyle and readiness to make changes, goal setting, dietary instruction, and evaluation.

C. To facilitate self care, the plan should be individualized and take into account cultural, lifestyle, and financial considerations. There is no "ADA diet," because the American Diabetes Association no longer endorses any single meal plan or specified percentages of macronutrients.

D. Focus should be on the total carbohydrates in the meals and eating a consistent amount of carbohydrate at each meal. Meal plans that prohibit concentrated sweets or are no sugar added, low sugar, or "liberal diabetic diets" only limit one type of carbohydrate (sugar) and are no longer appropriate.

E. Monitoring carbohydrate, whether by carbohydrate counting, choices, or experience-based estimation, remains a key strategy in achieving glycemic control.

F. Monitoring carbohydrate based on the glycemic index and glycemic load may provide an additional benefit over that observed when total carbohydrate is considered alone.

G. Monitoring of glucose and A1C, lipids, blood pressure, and renal status is essential to evaluate nutrition-related outcomes. If goals are not met, changes must be made in the overall diabetes care and management plan.

II. GOALS OF DIABETES MNT

A. Attain and maintain recommended metabolic outcomes, including glucose and A1C levels; LDL cholesterol, HDL cholesterol, and triglyceride levels; blood pressure; and body weight.

B. Prevent and treat the chronic complications and comorbidities of diabetes. Modify nutrient intake and lifestyle as appropriate for the prevention and treatment of obesity, dyslipidemia, CVD, hypertension, and nephropathy.

C. Improve health through healthful food choices and regular physical activity.

D. Address individual nutritional needs, taking into consideration personal and cultural beliefs and preferences and lifestyle while respecting the individual's wishes and willingness to change.

III. NUTRITIONAL RECOMMENDATIONS

A. Calories
  1. Intake necessary to achieve/maintain reasonable body weight, normal growth and development in children and adolescents, and increased needs during pregnancy and lactation or recovery from catabolic illness
  2. May require as little as 7% loss of body weight to achieve improved glycemic control
  3. In most cases a minimum of 1,200 kcal/day for women and 1,500 kcal/day for men are required to meet nutritional needs

B. Protein
  1. 10–20% of total daily calories is usual intake; 0.8–1.0 g/kg body weight/day for people with early stages of CKD; 0.8 g/kg body weight/day for those with later stages of CKD may improve measures of renal function.
  2. The long-term effects of >20% of daily dietary intake as protein on the development of nephropathy has not been determined.

C. Fat
  1. Amount based on nutrition assessment and treatment goals for glucose, lipids, and weight management
  2. Saturated fat intake <7% of calories
  3. Limit trans fats to lower LDL cholesterol and increase HDL cholesterol
  4. Fiber intake: 14g fiber/1,000 kcal) and increase consumption of whole grains to at least 1/2 of all grains

D. Carbohydrate (sugars, starches, soluble and insoluble fiber)
  1. The total amount of carbohydrate in meals and snacks is more important than the type.

E. Sodium: the goal is to reduce sodium intake to <1,500 mg per day for people with hypertension and <2,300 mg for all others.

F. Supplementation: Routine supplementation with antioxidants, such as vitamins E and C and carotene, is not advised because of lack of evidence of efficacy and concern related to long-term safety.

G. Alcohol
1. Drink alcohol only if diabetes is in good control and only in moderate amounts (limit one drink for women and two drinks for men per day).
2. Always consume food with alcohol. Drinking alcohol without food may cause hypoglycemia up to 24 hours later; risk is increased if taking insulin or insulin secretagogues.

IV. MNT GOALS FOR SPECIFIC SITUATIONS

A. For youth with type 1 diabetes, provide adequate energy to ensure normal growth and development; integrate insulin regimens into usual eating and physical activity habits.

B. For youth with type 2 diabetes, facilitate changes in eating and physical activity habits that reduce insulin resistance and improve metabolic status and encourage weight loss.

C. For pregnant and lactating women, provide adequate energy and nutrients needed for optimal outcomes.

D. For older adults, provide for the nutritional and psychosocial needs of an aging individual.

E. For individuals treated with insulin or insulin secretagogues, provide self-management education for treatment (and prevention) of hypoglycemia, acute illnesses, and exercise-related blood glucose problems.

F. For individuals at risk for diabetes, decrease risk by encouraging physical activity and promoting food choices that facilitate moderate weight loss or at least prevent weight gain.

G. For sick-day guidelines, see Illness (page 43).

H. For hospitalized patients:
1. Often only a nutritional assessment and provision of initial or basic nutrition education can be accomplished; diabetes nutrition self-management education is best provided in an outpatient or home setting.
2. Oral diabetes medications should be discontinued in favor of insulin to maintain metabolic control.

3. Patients with insulin deficiency (e.g., type 1 diabetes) must receive basal insulin despite reductions or absence of calorie intake to prevent diabetic ketoacidosis.

4. After surgery, food intake should be initiated as quickly as possible.

5. During catabolic illness, careful and continuous monitoring of nutritional and glycemic status is critical to ensure that increased nutritional needs are met and that hyperglycemia is prevented.

    a. Calorie needs for most patients are in the range of 25–35 kcal/kg every 24 hours, but should be individually determined.

    b. For patients with normal hepatic and renal function, protein needs are 1.0–1.5 g/kg body weight, depending on degree of stress.

6. Total grams of carbohydrate in enteral or parenteral formulations will have the greatest impact on glycemic response. A standard enteral feeding (50% carbohydrate) or a lower carbohydrate content formula (33–40% carbohydrate) may be used.

Exercise/Physical Activity

I. GOAL: A regular physical activity program, adapted to the presence of complications, is recommended for all patients with diabetes for general health benefits and weight loss. Regular physical activity reduces insulin resistance and can delay or prevent type 2 diabetes in high-risk individuals.

II. SAFETY GUIDELINES

A. Use clinical judgment in pre-exercise evaluation; patient age and previous physical activity level should be considered.

B. High risk patients should be encouraged to start with short periods of low-intensity exercise and increase the intensity and duration slowly.

C. Assess patients for conditions that might contraindicate certain types of exercise or predispose to injury, such as uncontrolled hypertension, severe autonomic neuropathy, severe peripheral neuropathy or history of foot lesions, and unstable proliferative retinopathy.

D. Monitor blood glucose levels to perceive patterns in glucose response and act to prevent hypoglycemia if using insulin or insulin secretagogue.
  1. Increase in body activity and temperature increases insulin action.
  2. Avoid exercising when insulin action peaking unless appropriate glucose availability.
  3. Option of decreasing pre-exercise insulin dose. Options include a 25–50% reduction of premeal bolus (for those on MDI or pumps), a temporary basal rate reduction (for those on pumps), and/or an extra 15 g carbohydrate uncovered with extra insulin for every 20 minutes or so of unusual exercise.
  4. Carry glucose tablets or gel.
  5. Exercise can lower glucose for up to 24 hours.
  6. Blood glucose <100 mg/dl (<5.5 mmol/l) before exercise. Eat 15 g carbohydrate, wait 15 minutes, and then check blood glucose again. Do not begin exercise until blood glucose >100 mg/dl.
  7. Blood glucose ≥250 mg/dl (≥13.9 mmol/l) with ketones, delay exercise until ketones negative. Treat immediately.

E. Monitor foot condition for signs of infection or ulcer if compromised sensitivity or vascular health. Instruct patient to wear comfortable clothing/footwear when exercising.

F. Wear medical identification indicating diabetes in a visible place.

G. Stop exercise if signs of overexertion or heart complications occur:
   1. Lightheadedness, dizziness
   2. Tightness in chest, fullness, heaviness, discomfort, or pain
   3. Severe or unusual shortness of breath
   4. Nausea

III. PERFORMANCE GUIDELINES

A. Individualize activity based on individual need, limitations, and personal preference.

B. Perform at least 150 minutes per week of moderate-intensity physical activity such as brisk walking.

C. Self-monitor target heart rate between 50 and 70% of estimated maximum heart rate (individualized to patient's resting heart rate).

D. In the absence of contraindications, people with type 2 diabetes should be encouraged to perform resistance training three times per week.

E. Patients with impaired glucose tolerance (IGT), impaired fasting glucose (IFG), or an A1C of 5.7–6.4% should be referred to an effective ongoing support program targeting weight loss of 7% of body weight and increasing physical activity.

Bariatric Surgery

I. GOAL: Meaningful weight loss in certain (severely) obese patients in whom lifestyle changes such as behavioral therapy, dietary modification, and exercise have not helped.

II. RECOMMENDATIONS

A. May be considered for adults with BMI ≥ 40 kg/m^2 or a BMI ≥ 35 kg/m^2 with type 2 diabetes, especially if the diabetes or other associated comorbidities are difficult to control with lifestyle and pharmacologic therapy.

B. Insufficient evidence to generally recommend surgery in patients with BMI <35 kg/m^2 outside of a research protocol.

C. Patients are usually discharged several days postoperatively and closely monitored for six weeks.

III. CONSIDERATIONS

A. Weight-loss surgeries have been shown to result in significant weight loss, as well as improvement in or remission of diabetes, roughly 80% of cases.

B. Diabetes patients are at increased risk of perioperative CV mortality, which needs to be evaluated and considered, especially in patients >50 years of age.

C. Favorable hormonal changes that can stimulate insulin secretion (after gastric bypass); glucose must be monitored closely after surgery.

D. Bariatric surgery is costly in the short term and has risks; associated risks can be reduced when procedure is performed by an experienced bariatric surgeon working in a Center of Excellence as certified by the American College of Surgeons or the American Society of Bariatric Surgeons.

E. Long-term studies remain limited in size and scope.

III. MAJOR FORMS OF BARIATRIC SURGERY WITH SOME ADVANTAGES AND DISADVANTAGES OF EACH PROCEDURE

Surgery	Strengths	Weaknesses
Roux-en-Y gastric bypass	• Most common form of bariatric surgery in the U.S. • Less malabsorptive than duodenal switch • Improvement in hypertension, hyperlipidemia, and diabetes	• More invasive than gastric banding • Malabsorption may lead to vitamin deficiencies • Higher risk of complications than gastric banding
Duodenal switch	• Highest rate of weight loss • Improvement in hypertension, hyperlipidemia, and diabetes	• Greatest risk of vitamin deficiencies • Greatest risk of complications
Gastric banding	• Smallest risk of complications • Least invasive procedure	• Least improvement in hyperlipidemia, hypertension, and diabetes

Foot and Skin Care

I. GOAL: Prevention, early detection of risk factors, and treatment of skin or foot problems caused by diabetes.

II. SKIN CARE RECOMMENDATIONS

One in three people with diabetes will have skin disorder caused or affected by diabetes in their lives. Skin problems can be first sign of diabetes.

A. Skin problems may include
   1. Bacterial infections (stye, foruncle, folliculitis, carbuncles, infections around the nails)
   2. Fungal infections
   3. Itching
   4. Diabetic dermopathy
   5. Necrobiosis lipoidica diabeticorum
   6. Diabetic blisters
   7. Eruptive xanthomatosis
   8. Acanthosis nigricans

B. Refer to dermatologist if indicated

C. Patient education
   1. Keep skin dry and clean
   2. Avoid very hot baths and showers
   3. Prevent dry skin
   4. Treat cuts right away
   5. During cold, dry months, use humidifier to add moisture; bathe less often
   6. Use mild shampoos
   7. See a dermatologist if skin problems persist
   8. Pay attention to foot health

III. FOOT CARE RECOMMENDATIONS

Limit morbidity and disability caused by diabetic ulcers and amputations. Daily foot care is essential in individuals with sensation loss due to peripheral neuropathy and/or peripheral arterial disease.

A. Annual foot exam
   1. Pedal pulses, history of claudication

2. Skin integrity (examining soles and between the toes)
3. Neurological status (vibratory sense), with somatosensory threshold testing with 10-g monofilament
4. Evidence of increased pressure:
    a. Erythema
    b. Warmth
    c. Hemorrhage under callus
5. Bony deformities
6. Limited joint mobility
7. Gait and balance
8. Ask about history of previous foot ulceration or amputation, neuropathic or peripheral vascular symptoms, impaired vision, tobacco use, and foot care practices.

B. **Patient education**
1. Smoking cessation
2. Optimize glucose control
3. Appropriate footwear to manage foot structure and biomechanics
4. Never go barefoot

	Signs	**Symptoms**
Vascular	Absent pedal or femoral pulses, femoral bruits	Cold feet, intermittent claudication of calf or foot pain at rest
Neurological	Sensory: reduced sensation to light touch, reduced pain and temperature perception	Sensory: burning, tingling, or crawling feelings; pain; hypersensitivity
	Motor: weakness	Motor: decreased deep-tendon reflexes
	Autonomic: decreased sweating	Autonomic: decreased sweating
Musculoskeletal	Claw toes, drop foot, "rocker bottom" feet	Gradual changes in foot shape, swelling without history of trauma
Dermatological	Skin: abnormal dryness, chronic infection, lesions and ulcers	Painless or painful wounds, slow-healing or nonhealing wounds, skin color changes, recurrent infections, chronic scaling and itching of dry feet
	Hair: decreased or absent	
	Nails: infection, ingrown nails, trophic changes, ulcerations or abscesses	

Stress Management/ Psychosocial Well-Being

I. GOAL: Improve wellbeing and coping skills. Stress, especially stress of illness, trauma, and/or surgery frequently aggravates glycemic control and may precipitate DKA or hyperglycemic hyperosmolar state, life-threatening conditions that require immediate medical care to prevent complications and death. Stress may also affect the onset of diabetes and is linked to other unhealthy behaviors.

II. RECOMMENDATIONS

A. Screen for psychosocial problems such as depression and diabetes-related distress, anxiety, eating disorders, and cognitive impairment when self-management is poor.

B. Identify life events in previous year that are stressors (e.g., financial worries, work-related stress, divorce, death of a loved one) as benchmark for ongoing or acute stress.

C. Encourage active stress management to:
- Remove or minimize the source of the stress when possible (time management, problem solving, or coping skills, etc.)
- Change the response to the stressful situation (adoption of relaxation techniques)
- Modify longer-term effects of stress

D. Refer to a mental health professional or behavioral based diabetes education program, as needed.

Immunizations

I. GOAL: Prevent illness and related hospital admissions, morbidity, and mortality related to influenza and pneumococcal disease. People with diabetes may be at increased risk of the bacteremic form of pneumococcal infection and have been reported to have a high risk of nosocomial bacteremia, which has a mortality rate as high as 50%.

A. Annual influenza vaccine to all patients with diabetes at least 6 months of age.

B. Administer pneumococcal polysaccharide vaccine to all diabetic patients ≥2 years of age.
  1. A one-time revaccination is recommended for individuals >64 years of age previously immunized when they were <65 years of age if the vaccine was administered >5 years ago.
  2. Other indications for repeat vaccination include nephrotic syndrome, chronic renal disease, and other immunocompromised states, such as after transplantation.

Glossary

C-peptide: a connecting peptide; when proinsulin is split, it yields insulin and C-peptide. Can be used as a measure of endogenous insulin production.

Dawn phenomenon: a modest increase in blood glucose level in the predawn hours that corresponds with natural rise in counterregulatory hormones (cortisol, growth hormone, epinephrine) and insulin deficiency.

Diabetic ketoacidosis (DKA): a life-threatening, but reversible complication characterized by severe disturbance of carbohydrate, protein, and fat metabolism that results from insulin deficiency.

Gestational diabetes mellitus (GDM): any degree of glucose intolerance with onset or first recognition during pregnancy. Usually diagnosed during the 24th to 28th week of pregnancy. Glucose tolerance often returns to normal (90%) after delivery. Patient (and baby) are at risk for future type 2 diabetes.

Glutamic acid decarboxylase (GAD): presence of antibodies directed against this enzyme indicates immune-mediated islet cell destruction that can result in type 1 diabetes.

Honeymoon period: within weeks after diagnosis of type 1 diabetes, there may be some recovery of β-cell function; consequently, exogenous insulin requirements often decrease for weeks to months.

Hyperosmolar hyperglycemic state (HHS): an acute episode of hyperglycemia more commonly occurring in elderly patients taking oral hypoglycemic agents. Mortality rate is high (12–41%).

Impaired fasting glucose (IFG): fasting glucose level ≥100 but <126 mg/dl (≥5 6 but <7.8 mmol/l). May be a risk factor for future diabetes and cardiovascular disease.

Impaired glucose tolerance (IGT): OGTT glucose level ≥140 mg/dl (≥7.8 mmol/l) and <200 mg/dl (<11.1 mmol/l) 2 hours post–glucose load. Many individuals with IGT are normoglycemic in their daily lives and manifest hyperglycemia only when challenged with the oral glucose load during an OGTT.

Islet-cell antibodies (ICAs): presence of ICAs indicates an autoimmune process that can lead to B-cell destruction resulting in type 1 diabetes.

Ketonemia: an excess of ketone bodies in the blood.

Oral glucose tolerance test (OGTT): timed glucose challenge.

Pre-diabetes: IFG or IGT or A1C 5.7–6.4%.

Resources

The American Diabetes Association
1701 North Beauregard Street
Alexandria, VA 22311
1-800-DIABETES (800-342-2383)
www.diabetes.org

American Academy of Nurse Practitioners (AANP)
AANP National Administrative Office
PO Box 12846
Austin, TX 78711
512-442-4262
www.aanp.org

The American Association of Clinical Endocrinologists
245 Riverside Avenue
Suite 200
Jacksonville, FL 32202
1-904-353-7878
www.aace.com

The American Association of Diabetes Educators
200 W. Madison Street, Suite 800
Chicago, IL 60606
1–800–338–3633 or 312–424–2426
Diabetes Educator Access Line: 1–800–TEAMUP4 (1–800–832–6874)
Email: aade@aadenet.org
www.diabeteseducator.org

National Diabetes Education Program
1 Diabetes Way
Bethesda, MD 20814–9692
1–800–438–5383
Email: ndep@mail.nih.gov
http://ndep.nih.gov

Bibliography

American Diabetes Association: Clinical Practice Recommendations. *Diabetes Care* 34 (Suppl. 1), Jan 2011. View at http://diabetes.org/professional

   List of Standards (Supplement page numbers)

   Standards of Medical Care in Diabetes—2011, p. S11
   Diagnosis and Classification of Diabetes Mellitus, p. S62
   Diabetes Care in the School and Day Care Setting, p. S70
   Diabetes Management in Correctional Institutions, p. S75
   Diabetes and Employment, p. S82
   Third-Party Reimbursement for Diabetes Care, Self-Management Education, and Supplies, p. S87
   National Standards for Diabetes Self-Management Education, p. S89

American Diabetes Association: *Diabetic Foot Ulcers and Amputations: Epidemiology, Pathogenesis, Assessment, and Prevention.* CD-ROM in Powerpoint. 2001.

American Diabetes Association: *Intensive Diabetes Management.* 4th ed. Wolfs-Dorf, J, Ed. 2009.

American Diabetes Association: *Medical Management of Type 1 Diabetes.* 5th ed. Bode B, Ed. 2008.

American Diabetes Association: *Medical Management of Type 2 Diabetes.* 6th ed. Burant C, Ed. 2008.

Antidiabetic agents. In *Drug Facts and Comparisons 2004.* St. Louis, MO, Wolters Kluwers, 2003, p. 357–388. Change to NPPR Nurse Practitioners' Prescribing Reference available at www.eMPR.com

Eckhauser AW, Richards WO, Fowler MJ. Bariatric surgery for patients with diabetes. *Clinical Diabetes* 25(3):83–89, 2007.

Endocrine Society Guidelines for Hyperglycemia Management in Hospitals. *Ann Intern Med*;154:260–267, 2011.

Clement S, Braithwaite SS, Magee MF, Ahmann A, Smith EP, Schager RG, Hirsch IB, on behalf of the Diabetes in Hospitals Writing Committee. Management of diabetes and hyperglycemia in hospitals (Technical Review). *Diabetes Care* 27:553–591, 2004.

Lloyd C, Smith J, Weinger K. Stress and diabetes: a review of the links. *Diabetes Spectrum* 18(2):121–127, 2005.

McNaughton CD, Self WH, Slovis C. Diabetes in the emergency department: acute care of diabetes patients. *Clinical Diabetes* 29(2):51–59, 2011.

Nathan DM, Buse JB, Davidson MB, Ferrannini et al. Medical management of hyperglycemia in type 2 diabetes: a consensus algorithm for theinitiation and adjustment of therapy: A consensus statement of the American Diabetes Association and the European Association for the Study of Diabetes. *Diabetes Care* 32(1):193–201, 2009.